POEMS ON THE BODY'S MESSENGERS

Sean Donnelly

Book Title Copyright © 2019 by Sean Donnelly. All Rights Reserved.

All rights reserved. No part of this book may be reproduced in any form or by any electronic or mechanical means including information storage and retrieval systems, without permission in writing from the author. The only exception is by a reviewer, who may quote short excerpts in a review.

Cover designed by Donna Canavan, Email: dbcbookproductions@gmail.com
About the Author photo by Jessica Snyder, Instagram: jesslaurenphoto@instagram

Sean's Poetry Collection, Book 2
Email: SeanDonnellyPoetry@gmail.com

Twitter: SeanDonnellyPoetry@poetry_sean
Facebook: https://www.facebook.com/Poems-on-the-Brain-332885280865871

Printed in the United States of America

Second Printing: Mar 2019
Amazon Kindle Direct Publishing

Book Description

Poetry you'll enjoy memorizing, science you'll learn easily. Click on the cover for a free preview! This book covers hormones and neurotransmitters, written to be beautiful to read and easy to comprehend. The formatting has been optimized for easy flashcard use between the title and the poem.

Science arose from poetry... when times change the two can meet again on a higher level as friends
—JOHANN WOLFGANG VON GOETHE

*For everyone who ever struggled in Chemistry because
they couldn't find the story.*

INTRODUCTION

This book began in 2018 while I was working on my first book Poems on the Brain. While reviewing the hormones and neurotransmitters that I really **should** cover, I recognized that I would need to write a wholly separate book just to cover those areas in depth. For one, there were too many to keep the length where I wanted. For two, many of these had action all over the body, and saying they just belonged to the brain would muddy the issue. So here goes!

Why you might want to read this book

If you enjoy poetry, this isn't the typical book du jour. It covers topics you'll be unlikely to discover anywhere else. This is fun because its new territory!

If you're studying the brain, you might enjoy this book because the poems are **designed** to be easily memorized. Each is actually a sestet (6 line poem) with the first line as the title of the chemical. The second line rhymes with it, and begins with the same letter, to make prompting recall easier.

If you're not one of the first two, you can still absolutely enjoy this book. A simple working knowledge of chemistry and biology are all you need to jump in. The emphasis is on the function, not the technical terms nor reactions.

What's changed with the format?

Previously, the format was also a 6 line poem, but the title of the anatomical structure (e.g. hypothalamus) wasn't part of the poem and it didn't rhyme. I made some changes to make these even easier. The poems now rhyme, with every 2 lines rhyming together. Additionally, the title at the top of the page **is** part of the poem now, and the second line will rhyme with it. This should help even more for folks attempting to remember the poems. Each line after the title is 8 syllables, up from the 6 in the previous book. Additionally, I've increased the font size at the bottom of the page for those who have trouble with small text. As always, I've kept the middle of the page empty so that folks can flashcard the top of the page versus the bottom. I've also added a couple pages at the end of the book for notes.

This had an effect on the preview poems from my previous book, Poems on the Brain (https://www.amazon.com/Poems-Brain-Sean-Donnelly-ebook/dp/B07H73YNYM). Since these were in the old format, I brought them up to date but kept the old ones as well, so that they could be enjoyed in both formats.

Caveat

I'm a poet writing about science. If you spot an error, please update me and I'll fix it in future editions. I plan to revise fairly regularly, as science is constantly changing and there is a real need to revisit the material and ensure accuracy for students.

Call to Action!

If you like this book- please review it so that others will see it. I preview poems from my future books on my Facebook page (https://www.facebook.com/Poems-on-the-Brain-332885280865871) for every review that I get.

I'd love to hear from my readership as well. Please make sure to send me an email if there's a poem you particularly enjoyed or a question that you have.

CONTENTS

INTRODUCTION 1
Format illustration: 7
Line 1 - Name of the Neurotransmitter/ Hormone 7
Acetylcholine 8
Adenosine 9
Adenosine Triphosphate 10
Adinopectin 11
Adrenocorticotropic hormone 12
Agouti-related peptide (AgRP) 13
Amylin (IAPP) 14
Anandamide 15
Angiotensin 16
Anti-Müllerian hormone (AMH) 17
Arginine 18
Aspartic Acid 19
Atrial natriuretic peptide (ANP) 20
Bradykinin 21
Calcitonin (thyrocalcitonin) 22
Cholecystokinin 24
Corticotropin-releasing hormone 25
Dehydroepiandrosterone (DHEA) 27
Dopamine 29
Endomorphin 30
Endorphin 31
Endothelin 32
Epinephrine 33
Erythropoietin 34
Estrogen (E) 35
Follicle Stimulating Hormone 36
Gamma-aminobutyricacid (GABA) 37

Gastrin	38
Ghrelin	39
Glucagon	40
Glutamic Acid	41
Glycine	42
Gonadotropin-reLeasing hormone (GnRH)	43
Growth Hormone Releasing Hormone (GHRH)	44
Hepcidin	45
Histamine	46
Human Growth Hormone	47
Hydrogen Sulfide	48
Insulin	49
Kisspeptin	50
Leptin	51
Luteinizing Hormone	52
Melatonin	53
Motilin	54
Neurokinin B (NKB)	55
Nitric Oxide	56
Norepinephrine	57
Orexin A	58
Oxytocin	59
Pancreatic Polypeptide	60
Peptide YY	61
Phenethylamine	62
Prolactin	63
Progesterone	64
Prostacyclin	65
Prostaglandins	66
Secretin	67
Serine	68
Serotonin	69
Somatostatin	70
Substance P	71
Testosterone (T)	72
Triiodothyronine	73
Tyramine	74
Vasoactive Intestinal Peptide (VIP)	75
Vasopressin	76
APPENDIX A: New Previews	78

Appendix B: Former Previews 85
Monoamine Neurotransmitters -Dopamine 86
Monoamine Neurotransmitters - Epinephrine (Adrenaline) 87
Monoamine Neurotransmitters - Histamine 88
Monoamine Neurotransmitters - Norepinephrine 89
Monoamine Neurotransmitters - Serotonin 90
About the Author 92
References 93
Notes 94
Notes 95

FORMAT ILLUSTRATION:

LINE 1 – NAME OF THE NEUROTRANSMITTER/ HORMONE

Line 2: rhymes with 1, word 1 starts with the same letter
Line 3: rhymes with 4
Line 4: rhymes with line 3
Line 5: rhymes with 6
Line 6: rhymes with line 5

ACETYLCHOLINE

Activate striated machine!
Turning on both nervous systems
Poison either excites or stems
The brain's ink for recollection
Nerve impulse and muscle flexion

ADENOSINE

Anti-arrhythmic from purine
When upper heart hastens heartbeat
If reentry, I may defeat
Turning off the heart's pacemaker
Opening blood-brain barrier

ADENOSINE TRIPHOSPHATE

Action currency, piece of eight
Covalent bonds store energy
Each glucose worth over thirty
With oxygen three parts convene
Phosphate, ribose, and adenine

ADINOPECTIN

Ably increased as you grow thin
Gluconeogenesis foil
Rewards with weight loss for your toil
Affecting brain through barrier
With leptin shrinks your derrière

ADRENOCORTICOTROPIC HORMONE

Abounding cortisol capstone
Supplied by pituitary
To adrenal cortex hurry
Securing cortisol's release
Stress and blood sugar to increase

AGOUTI-RELATED PEPTIDE (AGRP)

Aided weight gain may be relied
Stopped by leptin, helped by ghrelin
Your next weigh-in may cause chagrin
Stress and fasting increase my strength
Regaining all one's waistband length

AMYLIN (IAPP)

Accompanying insulin
Moderating glucose increase
When spiked causing hunger to cease
Diabetes Type 2 cell death
Vicious cycle, ever more strength

ANANDAMIDE

Antidepressant, bliss amide
Stopping the spread of breast cancer
Like THC (same receptor)
Black pepper halting re-uptake
Anxiety and fear to slake

ANGIOTENSIN

At peace with enzymes, though serpin
In four forms, I only makes II
Heightened blood pressure will ensue
Thirst, fat addition, kidney flow
Electrolyte and blood, winnow

ANTI-MÜLLERIAN HORMONE (AMH)

Active when male fetus present
Kills female reproductive tract
Each testis keeps its side intact
Wolffian male ducts built you see
Levels flip- flop at puberty

ARGININE

Ammonia bound for the latrine
Nitric oxide for blood pressure
Immune system T-cell booster
Made in intestines and kidneys
Essential in birds and babies

ASPARTIC ACID

Artificial sweetness tasted
Urea cycle donation
And goods for liquid absorption
Discovered in asparagus
At nitrogen uptake, peerless

ATRIAL NATRIURETIC PEPTIDE (ANP)

Atrium-made sodium guide
Opening mesangial cells
Sodium liberty compels
Calcium intrusion prevent
Averting heart-wall enlargement

BRADYKININ

Bequeathing venous dilation
Expansion dropping blood pressure
Bronchial and gut contractor
Espied by herpetologists
Pit viper venom it enlists

CALCITONIN (THYROCALCITONIN)

Calcium in blood reduction
Redepositing back in bone
Stopping mother's milk over-loan
Osteo-clast inhibition
So -blasts can fulfill their mission

CALCITRIOL

Calcium from food stockpile
Reabsorbing in renal tubes
When deficient, from bone removes
When in diet, good prognosis
Stopping osteoporosis

CHOLECYSTOKININ

Created in the intestine
Ordering digestive enzymes
And emptying gut take more time
Scarecrow in -4 causing panic
Parkinson's hallucinogenic

CORTICOTROPIN–RELEASING HORMONE

Creating, ACTH grown
Suicide and parturition
Nervous honing of attention
Major Depression, Alzheimer's
So stressed your hunger will disperse

Cortisol

Ceasing immune response to all
Through glucagon, blood sugar made
Glycogen, then muscle you trade
Stopping tissue inflammation
Slowed healing till stress cessation

DEHYDROEPIANDROSTERONE (DHEA)

Depending on sex, effect shown
Puberty's body hair and scent
In both, testosterones advent
Through DHT, hair loss in males
Made to estrogen in females

Dihydrotestosterone (DHT)

Directing male parts to be grown
Prostate and genitals mature
Baldness- something you may endure
From testosterone I'm derived
Male parts specific and short-lived

DOPAMINE

Drugs block my return to the scene
Predicting rewards will bring bliss
Overactive in psychosis
At low levels, pain will not cease
For nursing, stopping milk releas

ENDOMORPHIN

Ending pain, opioid akin
Holding onto urine, and breath
Strong analgesic unto death
K over Ca for relief
As always, excitation thief

ENDORPHIN

Endomorphin's strong, big brethren
We three: alpha, beta, gamma
Combined for analgesia
Morphine-like gamma making high
Running and laughter likewise pry

ENDOTHELIN

Elevate blood pressure within
Vasoconstriction sovereign
Atherosclerosis villain
Insulin resistance increased
Hypertension, soon be deceased

EPINEPHRINE

Excitement to prevent your end
Adrenals responding to fear
Fight or flight when danger is near
Used to treat Anaphylaxis
Heart stoppage and asthma dismiss

ERYTHROPOIETIN

Ensuring enough blood within
Guarding against hypoxia
Red blood cell building mania
Adult's mainly made in kidneys
Produced in liver by babies

ESTROGEN (E)

Estradiol- mating main one
Breasts, hips, and menstrual cycle
Growth spurt and bone closure, final
Plus testosterone, libido
Without either, lust torpedoed

FOLLICLE STIMULATING HORMONE

Flowering the egg cells when grown
In males, Sertoli activate
Prompting sperm growth to procreate
In females, granulosa grow
Follicle's egg cell set to sow

GAMMA-AMINOBUTYRICACID (GABA)

Guarding lest nerves be engrafted
Nor neurons over-swell the skull
Warning against flaccid muscle
What excites youths calms the adult
As from the cell chloride pours out

GASTRIN

Go gastric acid secretion!
For foods high protein and meaty
Three forms made: big-, little-, mini-
Emptying the bowels, then stomach
Stops at low pH, pre-havoc

GHRELIN

Gut hunger when no food within
As stomach stretches, no more made
As it empties fullness will fade
In thinner folks, a lower dose
In obese, hunger without close

GLUCAGON

Garrison when sugar is gone
Counter hormone to insulin
Ordering sugar creation
Islet of Langerhans A cells
Stopping blood sugar dizzy spells

GLUTAMIC ACID

Gain to food, umami added
Removing excess nitrogen
Needed for GABA creation
Rare D- form used in the liver
Taste for learning, brain exciter

GLYCINE

Generic grist to make protein
Found even in the depths of space
Food additive to sweeten taste
Cosmetic and fertilizer
Nerve inhibiting messenger

GONADOTROPIN-RELEASING HORMONE (GNRH)

Gregarious hormone capstone
Females acting suggestively
Mother's guard young aggressively
Filling males with peer aggression
Upon succeeding, profusion

GROWTH HORMONE RELEASING HORMONE (GHRH)

Growth hormone's secretagogue, known
Produced in hypothalamus
Yes we're growing, get on the bus!
Somatostatin enemy
Body growth pulsing painfully

HEPCIDIN

Hampering iron's journey in
Hepatic portal system blocked
And within macrophages locked
Stopping iron inundation
Abrogating all absorption

HISTAMINE

Headed to bed, sneezing machine
Faster rate for more alertness
But suppressing effects of stress
Though behind allergy attacks
Immune response and to relax

HUMAN GROWTH HORMONE

Huge amplification of bone
Anabolic, all tissue grows
At puberty adult height shows
Made within pituitary
In   excess,   acromegaly

HYDROGEN SULFIDE

How potassium means I chide
Smooth muscle into relaxing
Blood vessels into dilating
Devil's gas, a rancid cologne
Torpor causing smell of brimstone

INSULIN

Issued when sugar is within
Building fat, protecting muscle
Glucose into cells I hustle
In Type 2, my message not heard
In Type 1, beta cells interred

KISSPEPTIN

Kisses proclaimed Pennsylvanian
Leptin produced emissary
Starting the pituitary
GnRH stimulation
Activating menstruation

LEPTIN

Liquidating fat until thin
Fat cells signal to be consumed
By leptin's release, they are doomed
Though more is made in the obese
Unknown issues make message cease

LUTEINIZING HORMONE

Levels rise till follicle sewn
Raising testosterone in males
Pulsed unless GnRH fails
Setting the stage for conception
T-levels raised, lust inception

MELATONIN

Mobilizing you to sleep in
Expunging cell free radicals
Fighting immune system struggles
Found in grain and tannin plant foods
Made in third eye, with blue light feuds

MOTILIN

Motion through the gut I linchpin
At high pH, I start motion
At low, peristalsis is done
Ghrelin induced stomach cleaner
Somatostatin releaser

NEUROKININ B (NKB)

Neonate maturation key
Negative feedback cycle boost
GnRH and LH loosed
Preeclampsia when too high
With high blood pressure, both may die

NITRIC OXIDE

Needing greens to be satisfied
Free radical jumping membranes
With guanylate cyclase constrains
Calcium to vasodilate
Smooth muscle tension to abate

NOREPINEPHRINE

Needed for when troubles begin
Making glucose for energy
High blood pressure, in jeopardy
Located "alongside" kidneys
Telling cell maintenance to freeze

OREXIN A

Offering energy to play
Having eyes too big for your plate
Through me Tiredness to abate
In my absence, narcolepsy
Body fat and sleeping balance

OXYTOCIN

Orchestrating your next love-in
Mother-child, woman-to-man
Urging men to all others ban
Binding groups with food and grooming
Increasing trust and wound healing

PANCREATIC POLYPEPTIDE

Presents on blood-sugar downslide
Pancreatic arbitrator
Anorexia enabler
Controlling release of hormones
Until you are just skin and bones

PEPTIDE YY

Plump body fat will say goodbye
Release speed increased by fiber
Protein and nutrient binder
Appeasing hunger for weight loss
Body building, sloughing the dross

PHENETHYLAMINE

Physique alike monoamine
Euphoria and runner's high
Augmented by MAOI
Also stepped up by exercise
Stimulant with many likewise

PROLACTIN

Preparing milk for little one
Production-ready mammaries
Building fetal immunities
Suckling triggering milk-making
Oxytocin for thirst slaking

PROGESTERONE

Pregnancy preparing keystone
Readying uterus for sperm
For babe, immune system disarm
Pre-pregnancy, ovary-made
Later placenta will lend aid

PROSTACYCLIN

Platelet plug keeps blood in the tin
Does not occur while I'm present
Artificial used in treatment:
Ischemic blood supply to mend
And lung arteries reopened

PROSTAGLANDINS

Pain and blood control underpins
Inflates, dilates, loosens and clots
Not just one receptor, but lots
At COX, pain medications blocks
For when headache or fever knocks

SECRETIN

Setting water levels within
Leveraging stomach acid
Against bicarbonate pitted
Insulin made upon sweet taste
Carb and pH balance embraced

SERINE

Splitting enzymes, in poison seen
Nerve gases and insecticides
Rarity that we use D-sides
Normally only L speaker
Glycine and cysteine precursor

SEROTONIN

Stopping should my uptake begin
If it doesn't, making you high
Higher in a dominant guy
Controlling your pain and fullness
Wanting to action: coalesce

SOMATOSTATIN

Starting far or paracrine
Holding food within the stomach
Small intestine digestion stuck
Low pH acid controller
Human Growth Hormone aborter

SUBSTANCE P

Spanning cells omnipresently
Inflammation, nausea, and pain
Although healing, new flesh again
Warning of violence and poison
Body-protecting allergen

TESTOSTERONE (T)

Toughening up muscle and bone
Deep voice, fertility, and drive
Aggression and desire thrive
Spatial skills and sense of fair play
Romance and parenting belay

TRIIODOTHYRONINE

Three iodide Hormone machine
Pulse, eating, growth, and body heat
Metabolism made more fleet
Growing infant nerves, lungs and bones
Burning fat, turning abs to stones

TYRAMINE

Tyrant over monoamine
Pushing them out under my reign
Food causing wine-tasting migraine
From cocoa, wine, charcuterie
Smoked, aged, and fermented: tasty!

VASOACTIVE INTESTINAL PEPTIDE (VIP)

Vanguard hormone for the bedside
Vaginal and pancreatic
Bile, water, salt, and gastric
Secretions; and changed behavior
Circadian rhythm setter

VASOPRESSIN

Vouchsafes small bladder discipline
Anti-diuretic function
Having shape like oxytocin
Unknown effect on pair-bonding
Septic shock and bleed controlling

APPENDIX A: NEW PREVIEWS

From my new book, <u>Poems and Mistletoe</u>

MISTLETOE

Marriage on into Hades go
Poisoned arrow that killed Balder
Aeneas' underworld tour
Plucked berries, kisses under doors
Christmas kisses for new amours

SNOWFLAKES

Six-sided, unique, not mistakes
Singular beauty in many
Christ white as snow, shining brightly
Infinite shapes, number of man
Many in one, snow in snowman

WRAPPING PAPER

What's inside, colorful cypher
Delighting in the known unknown
Extravagant, or cheap cologne?
Colorful scenes of the season
Each day, delightful frustration

SWEATER WEATHER

Shivering at cold air, go burr!
Layers so the wind doesn't cut through
Woolen protection from the flu
Though some like to call them ugly
Green and red wears quite agelessly

CHRISTMAS TREE

Cut from ground or made chemically
Gratitude symbol, heart of home
Capped by angel or star at dome
Ornaments from previous years
Boniface stopping mother's tears

APPENDIX B: FORMER PREVIEWS

The 5 previews are reprinted here, for those who'd like to read them in their original format, from <u>Poems on the Brain.</u>

MONOAMINE NEUROTRANSMITTERS – DOPAMINE

Chemical messenger
Substantia nigra born
Action threshold setter
Too much brings psychosis
Too little causes pain
Impulsiveness benchmark

MONOAMINE NEUROTRANSMITTERS – EPINEPHRINE (ADRENALINE)

Adrenal gland produced
Fear induced secretion
No down-regulation
Memory enhancer
Berserker strength hormone
Fight or flight, get pumped up!

MONOAMINE NEUROTRANSMITTERS – HISTAMINE

Asleep versus awake
Set by rate of fire
Faster to be alert
Slower towards dreamland
Stimulating mucous
Sleepy and sneezing dwarves

MONOAMINE NEUROTRANSMITTERS – NOREPINEPHRINE

Sympathetic to stress
Maintenance to action
No sleep or digestion
Freeing up energy
To ensure survival
Vigilant defender

MONOAMINE NEUROTRANSMITTERS – SEROTONIN

5-HT receives me
Uptake stops my action
But if I'm left alone
Then I will get you high
Pain, fullness, and drug highs
Controller of good times

ABOUT THE AUTHOR

Sean Donnelly received his bachelors in Psychology and has taken numerous chemistry courses. He enjoys computer games (League of Legends, Overwatch, Heroes of the Storm, etc.) and loves to read textbooks. If you have enjoyed this book, he'd love to hear about it. He'd love a positive review on Amazon.com too. If he's wrong in any particular poem, he'd love to hear that too. Pending verification, he'll fix any errors/updates in the next edition. Thank you!

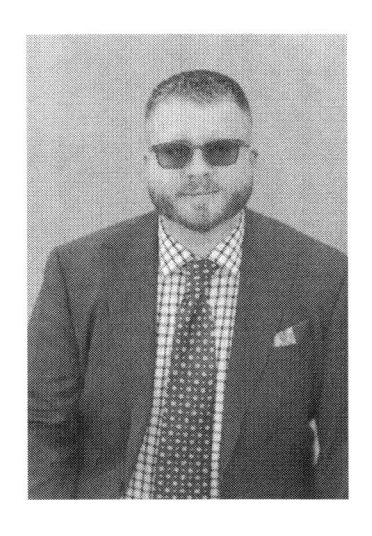

Email: SeanDonnellyPoetry@gmail.com

Facebook: https://www.facebook.com/Poems-on-the-Brain-332885280865871

Twitter: SeanDonnellyPoetry@poetry_sean

REFERENCES

Hall, J. E., & Guyton, A. C. (2006). *Textbook of Medical Physiology* (11th ed.). Philadelphia, PA: Saunders/Elsevier.

Kandel, E. R., Schwartz, J., & Jessell, T. (2000). *Principles of Neural Science* (4th ed.). NY, NY: McGraw-Hill Medical.

Main Page. (2019, January 28). Retrieved January 28, 2019, from https://www.wikipedia.org/

McMurry, J. (2000). *Organic Chemistry* (5th ed.). Pacific Grove, CA: Brooks Cole.

Neruda, P., & Tapscott, S. (2000). *100 Love Sonnets = Cien Sonetos de Amor*. Austin, TX: University of Texas Press.

Takemura, M., & Kikuyarō. (2009). *The Manga Guide to Biochemistry*. Tokyo, Japan: Ohmsha.

NOTES

NOTES

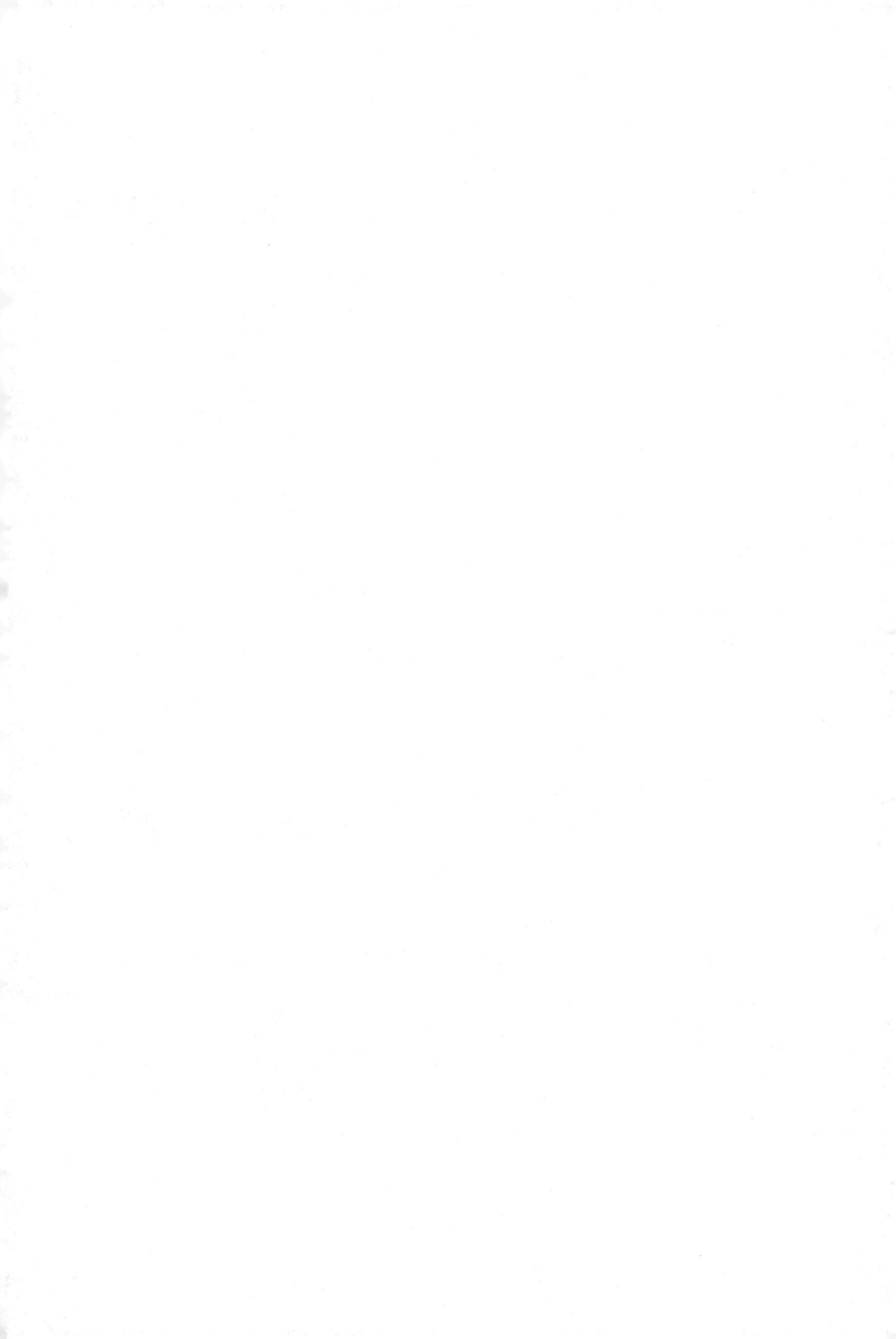

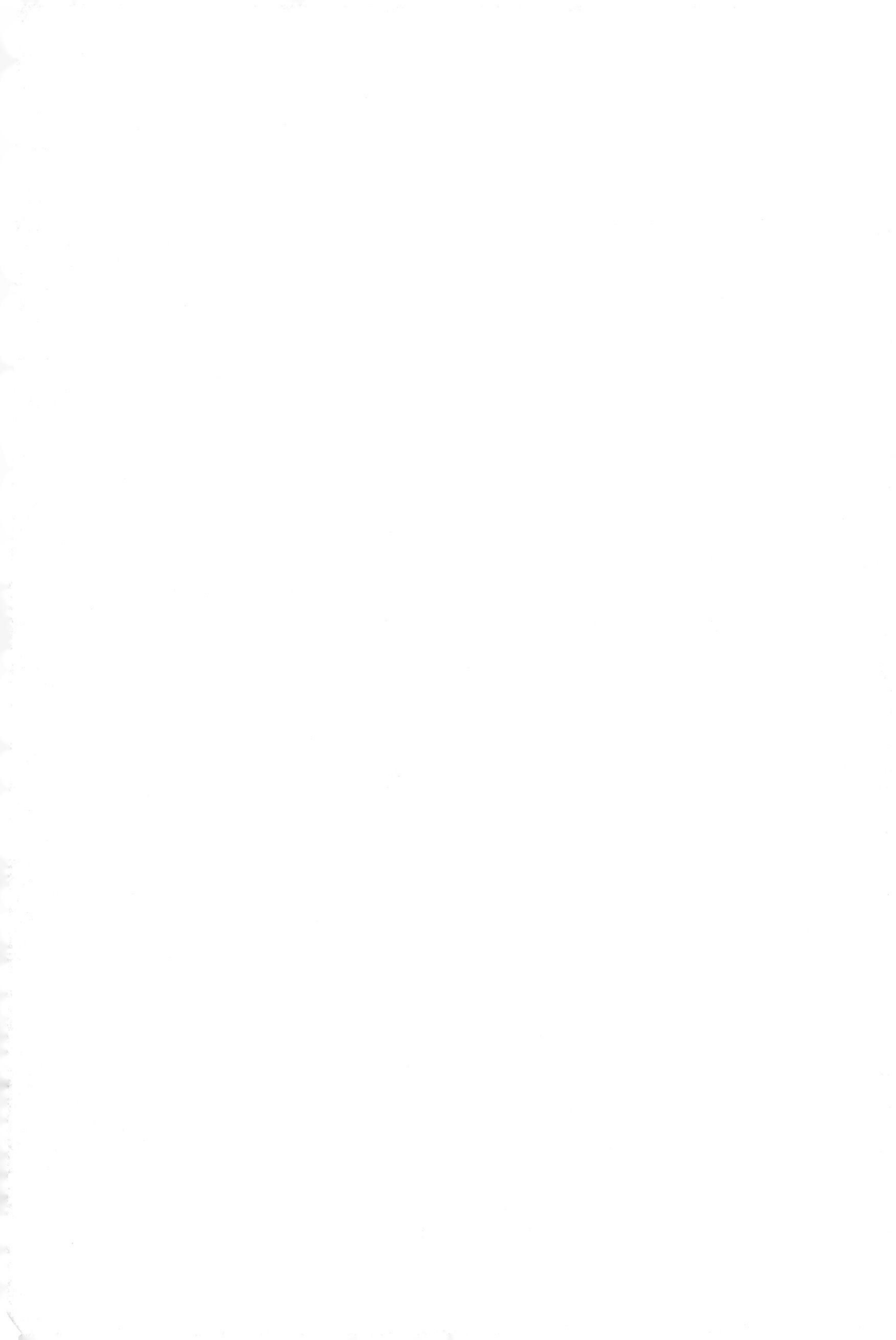

Made in the USA
Columbia, SC
06 May 2022